Big Print Diabetes Blood Sugar and Insulin Log

DATE:	INSULIN UNITS				BLOOD GLUCOSE READING						
	BREAKFAST	LUNCH	DINNER	EVENING	BREAKFAST	MID MORN	LUNCH	AFTERNOON	DINNER	EVENING	BEDTIME
MONDAY											
TUESDAY											
WEDNESDAY											
THURSDAY											
FRIDAY											
SATURDAY											
SUNDAY											

Writing Journal

Published by:
Berhampore Press
Wellington, NZ
BerhamporePress@gmail.com

ISBN-13:
978-1544663128

ISBN-10:
1544663129

DATE:	INSULIN UNITS				BLOOD GLUCOSE READING						
	BREAKFAST	LUNCH	DINNER	EVENING	BREAKFAST	MID MORN	LUNCH	AFTERNOON	DINNER	EVENING	BEDTIME
MONDAY											
TUESDAY											
WEDNESDAY											
THURSDAY											
FRIDAY											
SATURDAY											
SUNDAY											

NOTES

(Reasons for your blood glucose being high/low. Lack of exercise, sweets, carbs, alcohol etc.)

MONDAY:

TUESDAY:

WEDNESDAY:

THURSDAY:

FRIDAY:

SATURDAY:

SUNDAY:

DATE:	INSULIN UNITS				BLOOD GLUCOSE READING						
	BREAKFAST	LUNCH	DINNER	EVENING	BREAKFAST	MID MORN	LUNCH	AFTERNOON	DINNER	EVENING	BEDTIME
MONDAY											
TUESDAY											
WEDNESDAY											
THURSDAY											
FRIDAY											
SATURDAY											
SUNDAY											

NOTES

(Reasons for your blood glucose being high/low. Lack of exercise, sweets, carbs, alcohol etc.)

MONDAY:

TUESDAY:

WEDNESDAY:

THURSDAY:

FRIDAY:

SATURDAY:

SUNDAY:

DATE:	INSULIN UNITS				BLOOD GLUCOSE READING							
	B R E A K F A S T	L U N C H	D I N N E R	E V E N I N G	B R E A K F A S T	M I D M O R N	L U N C H	A F T E R N O O N	D I N N E R	E V E N I N G	B E D T I M E
MONDAY											
TUESDAY											
WEDNESDAY											
THURSDAY											
FRIDAY											
SATURDAY											
SUNDAY											

NOTES

(Reasons for your blood glucose being high/low. Lack of exercise, sweets, carbs, alcohol etc.)

MONDAY:

TUESDAY:

WEDNESDAY:

THURSDAY:

FRIDAY:

SATURDAY:

SUNDAY:

DATE:	INSULIN UNITS				BLOOD GLUCOSE READING						
	BREAKFAST	LUNCH	DINNER	EVENING	BREAKFAST	MID MORN	LUNCH	AFTERNOON	DINNER	EVENING	BEDTIME
MONDAY											
TUESDAY											
WEDNESDAY											
THURSDAY											
FRIDAY											
SATURDAY											
SUNDAY											

NOTES
(Reasons for your blood glucose being high/low. Lack of exercise, sweets, carbs, alcohol etc.)

MONDAY:

TUESDAY:

WEDNESDAY:

THURSDAY:

FRIDAY:

SATURDAY:

SUNDAY:

DATE:	INSULIN UNITS				BLOOD GLUCOSE READING						
	B R E A K F A S T	L U N C H	D I N N E R	E V E N I N G	B R E A K F A S T	M I D M O R N	L U N C H	A F T E R N O O N	D I N N E R	E V E N I N G	B E D T I M E
MONDAY											
TUESDAY											
WEDNESDAY											
THURSDAY											
FRIDAY											
SATURDAY											
SUNDAY											

NOTES
(Reasons for your blood glucose being high/low. Lack of exercise, sweets, carbs, alcohol etc.)

MONDAY:

TUESDAY:

WEDNESDAY:

THURSDAY:

FRIDAY:

SATURDAY:

SUNDAY:

DATE:	INSULIN UNITS				BLOOD GLUCOSE READING						
	BREAKFAST	LUNCH	DINNER	EVENING	BREAKFAST	MID MORN	LUNCH	AFTERNOON	DINNER	EVENING	BEDTIME
MONDAY											
TUESDAY											
WEDNESDAY											
THURSDAY											
FRIDAY											
SATURDAY											
SUNDAY											

NOTES
(Reasons for your blood glucose being high/low. Lack of exercise, sweets, carbs, alcohol etc.)

MONDAY:

TUESDAY:

WEDNESDAY:

THURSDAY:

FRIDAY:

SATURDAY:

SUNDAY:

DATE:	INSULIN UNITS				BLOOD GLUCOSE READING							
	BREAKFAST	LUNCH	DINNER	EVENING	BREAKFAST	MID MORN	LUNCH	AFTERNOON	DINNER	EVENING	BEDTIME	
MONDAY												
TUESDAY												
WEDNESDAY												
THURSDAY												
FRIDAY												
SATURDAY												
SUNDAY												

NOTES

(Reasons for your blood glucose being high/low. Lack of exercise, sweets, carbs, alcohol etc.)

MONDAY:

TUESDAY:

WEDNESDAY:

THURSDAY:

FRIDAY:

SATURDAY:

SUNDAY:

DATE:	INSULIN UNITS				BLOOD GLUCOSE READING							
	B R E A K F A S T	L U N C H	D I N N E R	E V E N I N G	B R E A K F A S T	M I D M O R N	L U N C H	A F T E R N O O N	D I N N E R	E V E N I N G	B E D T I M E	
MONDAY												
TUESDAY												
WEDNESDAY												
THURSDAY												
FRIDAY												
SATURDAY												
SUNDAY												

NOTES

(Reasons for your blood glucose being high/low. Lack of exercise, sweets, carbs, alcohol etc.)

MONDAY:

TUESDAY:

WEDNESDAY:

THURSDAY:

FRIDAY:

SATURDAY:

SUNDAY:

DATE:	INSULIN UNITS				BLOOD GLUCOSE READING						
	BREAKFAST	LUNCH	DINNER	EVENING	BREAKFAST	MID MORN	LUNCH	AFTERNOON	DINNER	EVENING	BEDTIME
MONDAY											
TUESDAY											
WEDNESDAY											
THURSDAY											
FRIDAY											
SATURDAY											
SUNDAY											

NOTES

(Reasons for your blood glucose being high/low. Lack of exercise, sweets, carbs, alcohol etc.)

MONDAY:

TUESDAY:

WEDNESDAY:

THURSDAY:

FRIDAY:

SATURDAY:

SUNDAY:

DATE:	INSULIN UNITS				BLOOD GLUCOSE READING							
	BREAKFAST	LUNCH	DINNER	EVENING	BREAKFAST	MID MORN	LUNCH	AFTERNOON	DINNER	EVENING	BEDTIME	
MONDAY												
TUESDAY												
WEDNESDAY												
THURSDAY												
FRIDAY												
SATURDAY												
SUNDAY												

NOTES
(Reasons for your blood glucose being high/low. Lack of exercise, sweets, carbs, alcohol etc.)

MONDAY:

TUESDAY:

WEDNESDAY:

THURSDAY:

FRIDAY:

SATURDAY:

SUNDAY:

DATE:	INSULIN UNITS				BLOOD GLUCOSE READING						
	BREAKFAST	LUNCH	DINNER	EVENING	BREAKFAST	MID MORN	LUNCH	AFTERNOON	DINNER	EVENING	BEDTIME
MONDAY											
TUESDAY											
WEDNESDAY											
THURSDAY											
FRIDAY											
SATURDAY											
SUNDAY											

NOTES
(Reasons for your blood glucose being high/low. Lack of exercise, sweets, carbs, alcohol etc.)

MONDAY:

TUESDAY:

WEDNESDAY:

THURSDAY:

FRIDAY:

SATURDAY:

SUNDAY:

DATE:	INSULIN UNITS				BLOOD GLUCOSE READING						
	BREAKFAST	LUNCH	DINNER	EVENING	BREAKFAST	MID MORN	LUNCH	AFTERNOON	DINNER	EVENING	BEDTIME
MONDAY											
TUESDAY											
WEDNESDAY											
THURSDAY											
FRIDAY											
SATURDAY											
SUNDAY											

NOTES
(Reasons for your blood glucose being high/low. Lack of exercise, sweets, carbs, alcohol etc.)

MONDAY:

TUESDAY:

WEDNESDAY:

THURSDAY:

FRIDAY:

SATURDAY:

SUNDAY:

DATE:	INSULIN UNITS				BLOOD GLUCOSE READING						
	BREAKFAST	LUNCH	DINNER	EVENING	BREAKFAST	MID MORN	LUNCH	AFTERNOON	DINNER	EVENING	BEDTIME
MONDAY											
TUESDAY											
WEDNESDAY											
THURSDAY											
FRIDAY											
SATURDAY											
SUNDAY											

NOTES

(Reasons for your blood glucose being high/low. Lack of exercise, sweets, carbs, alcohol etc.)

MONDAY:

TUESDAY:

WEDNESDAY:

THURSDAY:

FRIDAY:

SATURDAY:

SUNDAY:

DATE:	INSULIN UNITS				BLOOD GLUCOSE READING							
	BREAKFAST	LUNCH	DINNER	EVENING	BREAKFAST	MID MORN	LUNCH	AFTERNOON	DINNER	EVENING	BEDTIME
MONDAY											
TUESDAY											
WEDNESDAY											
THURSDAY											
FRIDAY											
SATURDAY											
SUNDAY											

NOTES

(Reasons for your blood glucose being high/low. Lack of exercise, sweets, carbs, alcohol etc.)

MONDAY:

TUESDAY:

WEDNESDAY:

THURSDAY:

FRIDAY:

SATURDAY:

SUNDAY:

DATE:		INSULIN UNITS				BLOOD GLUCOSE READING							
		BREAKFAST	LUNCH	DINNER	EVENING	BREAKFAST	MID MORN	LUNCH	AFTERNOON	DINNER	EVENING	BEDTIME
MONDAY												
TUESDAY												
WEDNESDAY												
THURSDAY												
FRIDAY												
SATURDAY												
SUNDAY												

NOTES
(Reasons for your blood glucose being high/low. Lack of exercise, sweets, carbs, alcohol etc.)

MONDAY:

TUESDAY:

WEDNESDAY:

THURSDAY:

FRIDAY:

SATURDAY:

SUNDAY:

DATE:	INSULIN UNITS				BLOOD GLUCOSE READING						
	BREAKFAST	LUNCH	DINNER	EVENING	BREAKFAST	MID MORN	LUNCH	AFTERNOON	DINNER	EVENING	BEDTIME
MONDAY											
TUESDAY											
WEDNESDAY											
THURSDAY											
FRIDAY											
SATURDAY											
SUNDAY											

NOTES

(Reasons for your blood glucose being high/low. Lack of exercise, sweets, carbs, alcohol etc.)

MONDAY:

TUESDAY:

WEDNESDAY:

THURSDAY:

FRIDAY:

SATURDAY:

SUNDAY:

DATE:	INSULIN UNITS				BLOOD GLUCOSE READING						
	BREAKFAST	LUNCH	DINNER	EVENING	BREAKFAST	MID MORN	LUNCH	AFTERNOON	DINNER	EVENING	BEDTIME
MONDAY											
TUESDAY											
WEDNESDAY											
THURSDAY											
FRIDAY											
SATURDAY											
SUNDAY											

NOTES

(Reasons for your blood glucose being high/low. Lack of exercise, sweets, carbs, alcohol etc.)

MONDAY:

TUESDAY:

WEDNESDAY:

THURSDAY:

FRIDAY:

SATURDAY:

SUNDAY:

DATE:	INSULIN UNITS				BLOOD GLUCOSE READING						
	BREAKFAST	LUNCH	DINNER	EVENING	BREAKFAST	MID MORN	LUNCH	AFTERNOON	DINNER	EVENING	BEDTIME
MONDAY											
TUESDAY											
WEDNESDAY											
THURSDAY											
FRIDAY											
SATURDAY											
SUNDAY											

NOTES
(Reasons for your blood glucose being high/low. Lack of exercise, sweets, carbs, alcohol etc.)

MONDAY:

TUESDAY:

WEDNESDAY:

THURSDAY:

FRIDAY:

SATURDAY:

SUNDAY:

DATE:	INSULIN UNITS				BLOOD GLUCOSE READING						
	BREAKFAST	LUNCH	DINNER	EVENING	BREAKFAST	MID MORN	LUNCH	AFTERNOON	DINNER	EVENING	BEDTIME
MONDAY											
TUESDAY											
WEDNESDAY											
THURSDAY											
FRIDAY											
SATURDAY											
SUNDAY											

NOTES

(Reasons for your blood glucose being high/low. Lack of exercise, sweets, carbs, alcohol etc.)

MONDAY:

TUESDAY:

WEDNESDAY:

THURSDAY:

FRIDAY:

SATURDAY:

SUNDAY:

DATE:	INSULIN UNITS				BLOOD GLUCOSE READING							
	BREAKFAST	LUNCH	DINNER	EVENING	BREAKFAST	MID MORN	LUNCH	AFTERNOON	DINNER	EVENING	BEDTIME
MONDAY											
TUESDAY											
WEDNESDAY											
THURSDAY											
FRIDAY											
SATURDAY											
SUNDAY											

NOTES

(Reasons for your blood glucose being high/low. Lack of exercise, sweets, carbs, alcohol etc.)

MONDAY:

TUESDAY:

WEDNESDAY:

THURSDAY:

FRIDAY:

SATURDAY:

SUNDAY:

DATE:	INSULIN UNITS				BLOOD GLUCOSE READING						
	BREAKFAST	LUNCH	DINNER	EVENING	BREAKFAST	MID MORN	LUNCH	AFTERNOON	DINNER	EVENING	BEDTIME
MONDAY											
TUESDAY											
WEDNESDAY											
THURSDAY											
FRIDAY											
SATURDAY											
SUNDAY											

NOTES

(Reasons for your blood glucose being high/low. Lack of exercise, sweets, carbs, alcohol etc.)

MONDAY:

TUESDAY:

WEDNESDAY:

THURSDAY:

FRIDAY:

SATURDAY:

SUNDAY:

DATE:	INSULIN UNITS				BLOOD GLUCOSE READING						
	BREAKFAST	LUNCH	DINNER	EVENING	BREAKFAST	MID MORN	LUNCH	AFTERNOON	DINNER	EVENING	BEDTIME
MONDAY											
TUESDAY											
WEDNESDAY											
THURSDAY											
FRIDAY											
SATURDAY											
SUNDAY											

NOTES

(Reasons for your blood glucose being high/low. Lack of exercise, sweets, carbs, alcohol etc.)

MONDAY:

TUESDAY:

WEDNESDAY:

THURSDAY:

FRIDAY:

SATURDAY:

SUNDAY:

DATE:	INSULIN UNITS				BLOOD GLUCOSE READING							
	BREAKFAST	LUNCH	DINNER	EVENING	BREAKFAST	MID MORN	LUNCH	AFTERNOON	DINNER	EVENING	BEDTIME
MONDAY											
TUESDAY											
WEDNESDAY											
THURSDAY											
FRIDAY											
SATURDAY											
SUNDAY											

NOTES
(Reasons for your blood glucose being high/low. Lack of exercise, sweets, carbs, alcohol etc.)

MONDAY:

TUESDAY:

WEDNESDAY:

THURSDAY:

FRIDAY:

SATURDAY:

SUNDAY:

DATE:	INSULIN UNITS				BLOOD GLUCOSE READING						
	BREAKFAST	LUNCH	DINNER	EVENING	BREAKFAST	MID MORN	LUNCH	AFTERNOON	DINNER	EVENING	BEDTIME
MONDAY											
TUESDAY											
WEDNESDAY											
THURSDAY											
FRIDAY											
SATURDAY											
SUNDAY											

NOTES
(Reasons for your blood glucose being high/low. Lack of exercise, sweets, carbs, alcohol etc.)

MONDAY:

TUESDAY:

WEDNESDAY:

THURSDAY:

FRIDAY:

SATURDAY:

SUNDAY:

DATE:	INSULIN UNITS				BLOOD GLUCOSE READING						
	BREAKFAST	LUNCH	DINNER	EVENING	BREAKFAST	MID MORN	LUNCH	AFTERNOON	DINNER	EVENING	BEDTIME
MONDAY											
TUESDAY											
WEDNESDAY											
THURSDAY											
FRIDAY											
SATURDAY											
SUNDAY											

NOTES
(Reasons for your blood glucose being high/low. Lack of exercise, sweets, carbs, alcohol etc.)

MONDAY:

TUESDAY:

WEDNESDAY:

THURSDAY:

FRIDAY:

SATURDAY:

SUNDAY:

DATE:	INSULIN UNITS				BLOOD GLUCOSE READING						
	B R E A K F A S T	L U N C H	D I N N E R	E V E N I N G	B R E A K F A S T	M I D M O R N	L U N C H	A F T E R N O O N	D I N N E R	E V E N I N G	B E D T I M E
MONDAY											
TUESDAY											
WEDNESDAY											
THURSDAY											
FRIDAY											
SATURDAY											
SUNDAY											

NOTES
(Reasons for your blood glucose being high/low. Lack of exercise, sweets, carbs, alcohol etc.)

MONDAY:

TUESDAY:

WEDNESDAY:

THURSDAY:

FRIDAY:

SATURDAY:

SUNDAY:

DATE:	INSULIN UNITS				BLOOD GLUCOSE READING						
	BREAKFAST	LUNCH	DINNER	EVENING	BREAKFAST	MID MORN	LUNCH	AFTERNOON	DINNER	EVENING	BEDTIME
MONDAY											
TUESDAY											
WEDNESDAY											
THURSDAY											
FRIDAY											
SATURDAY											
SUNDAY											

NOTES

(Reasons for your blood glucose being high/low. Lack of exercise, sweets, carbs, alcohol etc.)

MONDAY:

TUESDAY:

WEDNESDAY:

THURSDAY:

FRIDAY:

SATURDAY:

SUNDAY:

DATE:	INSULIN UNITS				BLOOD GLUCOSE READING						
	BREAKFAST	LUNCH	DINNER	EVENING	BREAKFAST	MID MORN	LUNCH	AFTERNOON	DINNER	EVENING	BEDTIME
MONDAY											
TUESDAY											
WEDNESDAY											
THURSDAY											
FRIDAY											
SATURDAY											
SUNDAY											

NOTES
(Reasons for your blood glucose being high/low. Lack of exercise, sweets, carbs, alcohol etc.)

MONDAY:

TUESDAY:

WEDNESDAY:

THURSDAY:

FRIDAY:

SATURDAY:

SUNDAY:

DATE:	INSULIN UNITS				BLOOD GLUCOSE READING						
	BREAKFAST	LUNCH	DINNER	EVENING	BREAKFAST	MID MORN	LUNCH	AFTERNOON	DINNER	EVENING	BEDTIME
MONDAY											
TUESDAY											
WEDNESDAY											
THURSDAY											
FRIDAY											
SATURDAY											
SUNDAY											

NOTES

(Reasons for your blood glucose being high/low. Lack of exercise, sweets, carbs, alcohol etc.)

MONDAY:

TUESDAY:

WEDNESDAY:

THURSDAY:

FRIDAY:

SATURDAY:

SUNDAY:

DATE:	INSULIN UNITS				BLOOD GLUCOSE READING						
	BREAKFAST	LUNCH	DINNER	EVENING	BREAKFAST	MID MORN	LUNCH	AFTERNOON	DINNER	EVENING	BEDTIME
MONDAY											
TUESDAY											
WEDNESDAY											
THURSDAY											
FRIDAY											
SATURDAY											
SUNDAY											

NOTES
(Reasons for your blood glucose being high/low. Lack of exercise, sweets, carbs, alcohol etc.)

MONDAY:

TUESDAY:

WEDNESDAY:

THURSDAY:

FRIDAY:

SATURDAY:

SUNDAY:

DATE:	INSULIN UNITS				BLOOD GLUCOSE READING						
	BREAKFAST	LUNCH	DINNER	EVENING	BREAKFAST	MID MORN	LUNCH	AFTERNOON	DINNER	EVENING	BEDTIME
MONDAY											
TUESDAY											
WEDNESDAY											
THURSDAY											
FRIDAY											
SATURDAY											
SUNDAY											

NOTES
(Reasons for your blood glucose being high/low. Lack of exercise, sweets, carbs, alcohol etc.)

MONDAY:

TUESDAY:

WEDNESDAY:

THURSDAY:

FRIDAY:

SATURDAY:

SUNDAY:

DATE:	INSULIN UNITS				BLOOD GLUCOSE READING						
	BREAKFAST	LUNCH	DINNER	EVENING	BREAKFAST	MID MORN	LUNCH	AFTERNOON	DINNER	EVENING	BEDTIME
MONDAY											
TUESDAY											
WEDNESDAY											
THURSDAY											
FRIDAY											
SATURDAY											
SUNDAY											

NOTES
(Reasons for your blood glucose being high/low. Lack of exercise, sweets, carbs, alcohol etc.)

MONDAY:

TUESDAY:

WEDNESDAY:

THURSDAY:

FRIDAY:

SATURDAY:

SUNDAY:

DATE:	INSULIN UNITS				BLOOD GLUCOSE READING						
	BREAKFAST	LUNCH	DINNER	EVENING	BREAKFAST	MID MORN	LUNCH	AFTERNOON	DINNER	EVENING	BEDTIME
MONDAY											
TUESDAY											
WEDNESDAY											
THURSDAY											
FRIDAY											
SATURDAY											
SUNDAY											

NOTES

(Reasons for your blood glucose being high/low. Lack of exercise, sweets, carbs, alcohol etc.)

MONDAY:

TUESDAY:

WEDNESDAY:

THURSDAY:

FRIDAY:

SATURDAY:

SUNDAY:

DATE:	INSULIN UNITS				BLOOD GLUCOSE READING						
	B R E A K F A S T	L U N C H	D I N N E R	E V E N I N G	B R E A K F A S T	M I D M O R N	L U N C H	A F T E R N O O N	D I N N E R	E V E N I N G	B E D T I M E
MONDAY											
TUESDAY											
WEDNESDAY											
THURSDAY											
FRIDAY											
SATURDAY											
SUNDAY											

NOTES
(Reasons for your blood glucose being high/low. Lack of exercise, sweets, carbs, alcohol etc.)

MONDAY:

TUESDAY:

WEDNESDAY:

THURSDAY:

FRIDAY:

SATURDAY:

SUNDAY:

DATE:	INSULIN UNITS				BLOOD GLUCOSE READING						
	B R E A K F A S T	L U N C H	D I N N E R	E V E N I N G	B R E A K F A S T	M I D M O R N	L U N C H	A F T E R N O O N	D I N N E R	E V E N I N G	B E D T I M E
MONDAY											
TUESDAY											
WEDNESDAY											
THURSDAY											
FRIDAY											
SATURDAY											
SUNDAY											

NOTES
(Reasons for your blood glucose being high/low. Lack of exercise, sweets, carbs, alcohol etc.)

MONDAY:

TUESDAY:

WEDNESDAY:

THURSDAY:

FRIDAY:

SATURDAY:

SUNDAY:

DATE:	INSULIN UNITS				BLOOD GLUCOSE READING							
	BREAKFAST	LUNCH	DINNER	EVENING	BREAKFAST	MID MORN	LUNCH	AFTERNOON	DINNER	EVENING	BEDTIME
MONDAY											
TUESDAY											
WEDNESDAY											
THURSDAY											
FRIDAY											
SATURDAY											
SUNDAY											

NOTES

(Reasons for your blood glucose being high/low. Lack of exercise, sweets, carbs, alcohol etc.)

MONDAY:

TUESDAY:

WEDNESDAY:

THURSDAY:

FRIDAY:

SATURDAY:

SUNDAY:

DATE:	INSULIN UNITS				BLOOD GLUCOSE READING						
	BREAKFAST	LUNCH	DINNER	EVENING	BREAKFAST	MID MORN	LUNCH	AFTERNOON	DINNER	EVENING	BEDTIME
MONDAY											
TUESDAY											
WEDNESDAY											
THURSDAY											
FRIDAY											
SATURDAY											
SUNDAY											

NOTES
(Reasons for your blood glucose being high/low. Lack of exercise, sweets, carbs, alcohol etc.)

MONDAY:

TUESDAY:

WEDNESDAY:

THURSDAY:

FRIDAY:

SATURDAY:

SUNDAY:

DATE:	INSULIN UNITS				BLOOD GLUCOSE READING							
	BREAKFAST	LUNCH	DINNER	EVENING	BREAKFAST	MID MORN	LUNCH	AFTERNOON	DINNER	EVENING	BEDTIME
MONDAY											
TUESDAY											
WEDNESDAY											
THURSDAY											
FRIDAY											
SATURDAY											
SUNDAY											

NOTES

(Reasons for your blood glucose being high/low. Lack of exercise, sweets, carbs, alcohol etc.)

MONDAY:

TUESDAY:

WEDNESDAY:

THURSDAY:

FRIDAY:

SATURDAY:

SUNDAY:

DATE:	INSULIN UNITS				BLOOD GLUCOSE READING						
	BREAKFAST	LUNCH	DINNER	EVENING	BREAKFAST	MID MORN	LUNCH	AFTERNOON	DINNER	EVENING	BEDTIME
MONDAY											
TUESDAY											
WEDNESDAY											
THURSDAY											
FRIDAY											
SATURDAY											
SUNDAY											

NOTES

(Reasons for your blood glucose being high/low. Lack of exercise, sweets, carbs, alcohol etc.)

MONDAY:

TUESDAY:

WEDNESDAY:

THURSDAY:

FRIDAY:

SATURDAY:

SUNDAY:

DATE:	INSULIN UNITS				BLOOD GLUCOSE READING						
	BREAKFAST	LUNCH	DINNER	EVENING	BREAKFAST	MID MORN	LUNCH	AFTERNOON	DINNER	EVENING	BEDTIME
MONDAY											
TUESDAY											
WEDNESDAY											
THURSDAY											
FRIDAY											
SATURDAY											
SUNDAY											

NOTES
(Reasons for your blood glucose being high/low. Lack of exercise, sweets, carbs, alcohol etc.)

MONDAY:

TUESDAY:

WEDNESDAY:

THURSDAY:

FRIDAY:

SATURDAY:

SUNDAY:

DATE:	INSULIN UNITS				BLOOD GLUCOSE READING						
	BREAKFAST	LUNCH	DINNER	EVENING	BREAKFAST	MID MORN	LUNCH	AFTERNOON	DINNER	EVENING	BEDTIME
MONDAY											
TUESDAY											
WEDNESDAY											
THURSDAY											
FRIDAY											
SATURDAY											
SUNDAY											

NOTES

(Reasons for your blood glucose being high/low. Lack of exercise, sweets, carbs, alcohol etc.)

MONDAY:

TUESDAY:

WEDNESDAY:

THURSDAY:

FRIDAY:

SATURDAY:

SUNDAY:

DATE:	INSULIN UNITS				BLOOD GLUCOSE READING						
	BREAKFAST	LUNCH	DINNER	EVENING	BREAKFAST	MID MORN	LUNCH	AFTERNOON	DINNER	EVENING	BEDTIME
MONDAY											
TUESDAY											
WEDNESDAY											
THURSDAY											
FRIDAY											
SATURDAY											
SUNDAY											

NOTES

(Reasons for your blood glucose being high/low. Lack of exercise, sweets, carbs, alcohol etc.)

MONDAY:

TUESDAY:

WEDNESDAY:

THURSDAY:

FRIDAY:

SATURDAY:

SUNDAY:

DATE:	INSULIN UNITS				BLOOD GLUCOSE READING						
	BREAKFAST	LUNCH	DINNER	EVENING	BREAKFAST	MID MORN	LUNCH	AFTERNOON	DINNER	EVENING	BEDTIME
MONDAY											
TUESDAY											
WEDNESDAY											
THURSDAY											
FRIDAY											
SATURDAY											
SUNDAY											

NOTES
(Reasons for your blood glucose being high/low. Lack of exercise, sweets, carbs, alcohol etc.)

MONDAY:

TUESDAY:

WEDNESDAY:

THURSDAY:

FRIDAY:

SATURDAY:

SUNDAY:

DATE:	INSULIN UNITS				BLOOD GLUCOSE READING						
	BREAKFAST	LUNCH	DINNER	EVENING	BREAKFAST	MID MORN	LUNCH	AFTERNOON	DINNER	EVENING	BEDTIME
MONDAY											
TUESDAY											
WEDNESDAY											
THURSDAY											
FRIDAY											
SATURDAY											
SUNDAY											

NOTES

(Reasons for your blood glucose being high/low. Lack of exercise, sweets, carbs, alcohol etc.)

MONDAY:

TUESDAY:

WEDNESDAY:

THURSDAY:

FRIDAY:

SATURDAY:

SUNDAY:

DATE:	INSULIN UNITS				BLOOD GLUCOSE READING						
	BREAKFAST	LUNCH	DINNER	EVENING	BREAKFAST	MID MORN	LUNCH	AFTERNOON	DINNER	EVENING	BEDTIME
MONDAY											
TUESDAY											
WEDNESDAY											
THURSDAY											
FRIDAY											
SATURDAY											
SUNDAY											

NOTES
(Reasons for your blood glucose being high/low. Lack of exercise, sweets, carbs, alcohol etc.)

MONDAY:

TUESDAY:

WEDNESDAY:

THURSDAY:

FRIDAY:

SATURDAY:

SUNDAY:

DATE:	INSULIN UNITS				BLOOD GLUCOSE READING						
	BREAKFAST	LUNCH	DINNER	EVENING	BREAKFAST	MID MORN	LUNCH	AFTERNOON	DINNER	EVENING	BEDTIME
MONDAY											
TUESDAY											
WEDNESDAY											
THURSDAY											
FRIDAY											
SATURDAY											
SUNDAY											

NOTES
(Reasons for your blood glucose being high/low. Lack of exercise, sweets, carbs, alcohol etc.)

MONDAY:

TUESDAY:

WEDNESDAY:

THURSDAY:

FRIDAY:

SATURDAY:

SUNDAY:

DATE:	INSULIN UNITS				BLOOD GLUCOSE READING						
	B R E A K F A S T	L U N C H	D I N N E R	E V E N I N G	B R E A K F A S T	M I D M O R N	L U N C H	A F T E R N O O N	D I N N E R	E V E N I N G	B E D T I M E
MONDAY											
TUESDAY											
WEDNESDAY											
THURSDAY											
FRIDAY											
SATURDAY											
SUNDAY											

NOTES
(Reasons for your blood glucose being high/low. Lack of exercise, sweets, carbs, alcohol etc.)

MONDAY:

TUESDAY:

WEDNESDAY:

THURSDAY:

FRIDAY:

SATURDAY:

SUNDAY:

DATE:	INSULIN UNITS				BLOOD GLUCOSE READING							
	BREAKFAST	LUNCH	DINNER	EVENING	BREAKFAST	MID MORN	LUNCH	AFTERNOON	DINNER	EVENING	BEDTIME
MONDAY											
TUESDAY											
WEDNESDAY											
THURSDAY											
FRIDAY											
SATURDAY											
SUNDAY											

NOTES

(Reasons for your blood glucose being high/low. Lack of exercise, sweets, carbs, alcohol etc.)

MONDAY:

TUESDAY:

WEDNESDAY:

THURSDAY:

FRIDAY:

SATURDAY:

SUNDAY:

DATE:	INSULIN UNITS				BLOOD GLUCOSE READING						
	BREAKFAST	LUNCH	DINNER	EVENING	BREAKFAST	MID MORN	LUNCH	AFTERNOON	DINNER	EVENING	BEDTIME
MONDAY											
TUESDAY											
WEDNESDAY											
THURSDAY											
FRIDAY											
SATURDAY											
SUNDAY											

NOTES
(Reasons for your blood glucose being high/low. Lack of exercise, sweets, carbs, alcohol etc.)

MONDAY:

TUESDAY:

WEDNESDAY:

THURSDAY:

FRIDAY:

SATURDAY:

SUNDAY:

DATE:	INSULIN UNITS				BLOOD GLUCOSE READING							
	BREAKFAST	LUNCH	DINNER	EVENING	BREAKFAST	MID MORN	LUNCH	AFTERNOON	DINNER	EVENING	BEDTIME
MONDAY											
TUESDAY											
WEDNESDAY											
THURSDAY											
FRIDAY											
SATURDAY											
SUNDAY											

NOTES

(Reasons for your blood glucose being high/low. Lack of exercise, sweets, carbs, alcohol etc.)

MONDAY:

TUESDAY:

WEDNESDAY:

THURSDAY:

FRIDAY:

SATURDAY:

SUNDAY:

DATE:	INSULIN UNITS				BLOOD GLUCOSE READING						
	BREAKFAST	LUNCH	DINNER	EVENING	BREAKFAST	MID MORN	LUNCH	AFTERNOON	DINNER	EVENING	BEDTIME
MONDAY											
TUESDAY											
WEDNESDAY											
THURSDAY											
FRIDAY											
SATURDAY											
SUNDAY											

NOTES

(Reasons for your blood glucose being high/low. Lack of exercise, sweets, carbs, alcohol etc.)

MONDAY:

TUESDAY:

WEDNESDAY:

THURSDAY:

FRIDAY:

SATURDAY:

SUNDAY:

DATE:	INSULIN UNITS				BLOOD GLUCOSE READING							
	BREAKFAST	LUNCH	DINNER	EVENING	BREAKFAST	MID MORN	LUNCH	AFTERNOON	DINNER	EVENING	BEDTIME
MONDAY											
TUESDAY											
WEDNESDAY											
THURSDAY											
FRIDAY											
SATURDAY											
SUNDAY											

NOTES
(Reasons for your blood glucose being high/low. Lack of exercise, sweets, carbs, alcohol etc.)

MONDAY:

TUESDAY:

WEDNESDAY:

THURSDAY:

FRIDAY:

SATURDAY:

SUNDAY:

DATE:	INSULIN UNITS				BLOOD GLUCOSE READING							
	BREAKFAST	LUNCH	DINNER	EVENING	BREAKFAST	MID MORN	LUNCH	AFTERNOON	DINNER	EVENING	BEDTIME
MONDAY											
TUESDAY											
WEDNESDAY											
THURSDAY											
FRIDAY											
SATURDAY											
SUNDAY											

NOTES
(Reasons for your blood glucose being high/low. Lack of exercise, sweets, carbs, alcohol etc.)

MONDAY:

TUESDAY:

WEDNESDAY:

THURSDAY:

FRIDAY:

SATURDAY:

SUNDAY:

DATE:	INSULIN UNITS				BLOOD GLUCOSE READING							
	BREAKFAST	LUNCH	DINNER	EVENING	BREAKFAST	MID MORN	LUNCH	AFTERNOON	DINNER	EVENING	BEDTIME
MONDAY											
TUESDAY											
WEDNESDAY											
THURSDAY											
FRIDAY											
SATURDAY											
SUNDAY											

NOTES

(Reasons for your blood glucose being high/low. Lack of exercise, sweets, carbs, alcohol etc.)

MONDAY:

TUESDAY:

WEDNESDAY:

THURSDAY:

FRIDAY:

SATURDAY:

SUNDAY:

DATE:	INSULIN UNITS				BLOOD GLUCOSE READING						
	BREAKFAST	LUNCH	DINNER	EVENING	BREAKFAST	MID MORN	LUNCH	AFTERNOON	DINNER	EVENING	BEDTIME
MONDAY											
TUESDAY											
WEDNESDAY											
THURSDAY											
FRIDAY											
SATURDAY											
SUNDAY											

NOTES
(Reasons for your blood glucose being high/low. Lack of exercise, sweets, carbs, alcohol etc.)

MONDAY:

TUESDAY:

WEDNESDAY:

THURSDAY:

FRIDAY:

SATURDAY:

SUNDAY:

DATE:	INSULIN UNITS				BLOOD GLUCOSE READING						
	BREAKFAST	LUNCH	DINNER	EVENING	BREAKFAST	MID MORN	LUNCH	AFTERNOON	DINNER	EVENING	BEDTIME
MONDAY											
TUESDAY											
WEDNESDAY											
THURSDAY											
FRIDAY											
SATURDAY											
SUNDAY											

NOTES

(Reasons for your blood glucose being high/low. Lack of exercise, sweets, carbs, alcohol etc.)

MONDAY:

TUESDAY:

WEDNESDAY:

THURSDAY:

FRIDAY:

SATURDAY:

SUNDAY:

DATE:	INSULIN UNITS				BLOOD GLUCOSE READING							
	B R E A K F A S T	L U N C H	D I N N E R	E V E N I N G	B R E A K F A S T	M I D M O R N	L U N C H	A F T E R N O O N	D I N N E R	E V E N I N G	B E D T I M E
MONDAY											
TUESDAY											
WEDNESDAY											
THURSDAY											
FRIDAY											
SATURDAY											
SUNDAY											

NOTES
(Reasons for your blood glucose being high/low. Lack of exercise, sweets, carbs, alcohol etc.)

MONDAY:

TUESDAY:

WEDNESDAY:

THURSDAY:

FRIDAY:

SATURDAY:

SUNDAY:

DATE:	INSULIN UNITS				BLOOD GLUCOSE READING							
	BREAKFAST	LUNCH	DINNER	EVENING	BREAKFAST	MID MORN	LUNCH	AFTERNOON	DINNER	EVENING	BEDTIME
MONDAY											
TUESDAY											
WEDNESDAY											
THURSDAY											
FRIDAY											
SATURDAY											
SUNDAY											

NOTES

(Reasons for your blood glucose being high/low. Lack of exercise, sweets, carbs, alcohol etc.)

MONDAY:

TUESDAY:

WEDNESDAY:

THURSDAY:

FRIDAY:

SATURDAY:

SUNDAY:

DATE:	INSULIN UNITS				BLOOD GLUCOSE READING						
	BREAKFAST	LUNCH	DINNER	EVENING	BREAKFAST	MID MORN	LUNCH	AFTERNOON	DINNER	EVENING	BEDTIME
MONDAY											
TUESDAY											
WEDNESDAY											
THURSDAY											
FRIDAY											
SATURDAY											
SUNDAY											

NOTES
(Reasons for your blood glucose being high/low. Lack of exercise, sweets, carbs, alcohol etc.)

MONDAY:

TUESDAY:

WEDNESDAY:

THURSDAY:

FRIDAY:

SATURDAY:

SUNDAY:

DATE:	INSULIN UNITS				BLOOD GLUCOSE READING							
	BREAKFAST	LUNCH	DINNER	EVENING	BREAKFAST	MID MORN	LUNCH	AFTERNOON	DINNER	EVENING	BEDTIME
MONDAY											
TUESDAY											
WEDNESDAY											
THURSDAY											
FRIDAY											
SATURDAY											
SUNDAY											

NOTES
(Reasons for your blood glucose being high/low. Lack of exercise, sweets, carbs, alcohol etc.)

MONDAY:

TUESDAY:

WEDNESDAY:

THURSDAY:

FRIDAY:

SATURDAY:

SUNDAY:

DATE:	INSULIN UNITS				BLOOD GLUCOSE READING							
	B R E A K F A S T	L U N C H	D I N N E R	E V E N I N G	B R E A K F A S T	M I D M O R N	L U N C H	A F T E R N O O N	D I N N E R	E V E N I N G	B E D T I M E
MONDAY											
TUESDAY											
WEDNESDAY											
THURSDAY											
FRIDAY											
SATURDAY											
SUNDAY											

NOTES
(Reasons for your blood glucose being high/low. Lack of exercise, sweets, carbs, alcohol etc.)

MONDAY:

TUESDAY:

WEDNESDAY:

THURSDAY:

FRIDAY:

SATURDAY:

SUNDAY:

DATE:	INSULIN UNITS				BLOOD GLUCOSE READING						
	BREAKFAST	LUNCH	DINNER	EVENING	BREAKFAST	MID MORN	LUNCH	AFTERNOON	DINNER	EVENING	BEDTIME
MONDAY											
TUESDAY											
WEDNESDAY											
THURSDAY											
FRIDAY											
SATURDAY											
SUNDAY											

NOTES

(Reasons for your blood glucose being high/low. Lack of exercise, sweets, carbs, alcohol etc.)

MONDAY:

TUESDAY:

WEDNESDAY:

THURSDAY:

FRIDAY:

SATURDAY:

SUNDAY:

DATE:		INSULIN UNITS				BLOOD GLUCOSE READING							
		BREAKFAST	LUNCH	DINNER	EVENING	BREAKFAST	MID MORN	LUNCH	AFTERNOON	DINNER	EVENING	BEDTIME
MONDAY												
TUESDAY												
WEDNESDAY												
THURSDAY												
FRIDAY												
SATURDAY												
SUNDAY												

NOTES
(Reasons for your blood glucose being high/low. Lack of exercise, sweets, carbs, alcohol etc.)

MONDAY:

TUESDAY:

WEDNESDAY:

THURSDAY:

FRIDAY:

SATURDAY:

SUNDAY:

DATE:	INSULIN UNITS				BLOOD GLUCOSE READING						
	BREAKFAST	LUNCH	DINNER	EVENING	BREAKFAST	MID MORN	LUNCH	AFTERNOON	DINNER	EVENING	BEDTIME
MONDAY											
TUESDAY											
WEDNESDAY											
THURSDAY											
FRIDAY											
SATURDAY											
SUNDAY											

NOTES
(Reasons for your blood glucose being high/low. Lack of exercise, sweets, carbs, alcohol etc.)

MONDAY:

TUESDAY:

WEDNESDAY:

THURSDAY:

FRIDAY:

SATURDAY:

SUNDAY:

DATE:	INSULIN UNITS				BLOOD GLUCOSE READING						
	BREAKFAST	LUNCH	DINNER	EVENING	BREAKFAST	MID MORN	LUNCH	AFTERNOON	DINNER	EVENING	BEDTIME
MONDAY											
TUESDAY											
WEDNESDAY											
THURSDAY											
FRIDAY											
SATURDAY											
SUNDAY											

NOTES

(Reasons for your blood glucose being high/low. Lack of exercise, sweets, carbs, alcohol etc.)

MONDAY:

TUESDAY:

WEDNESDAY:

THURSDAY:

FRIDAY:

SATURDAY:

SUNDAY:

DATE:	INSULIN UNITS				BLOOD GLUCOSE READING						
	BREAKFAST	LUNCH	DINNER	EVENING	BREAKFAST	MID MORN	LUNCH	AFTERNOON	DINNER	EVENING	BEDTIME
MONDAY											
TUESDAY											
WEDNESDAY											
THURSDAY											
FRIDAY											
SATURDAY											
SUNDAY											

NOTES

(Reasons for your blood glucose being high/low. Lack of exercise, sweets, carbs, alcohol etc.)

MONDAY:

TUESDAY:

WEDNESDAY:

THURSDAY:

FRIDAY:

SATURDAY:

SUNDAY:

DATE:	INSULIN UNITS				BLOOD GLUCOSE READING						
	BREAKFAST	LUNCH	DINNER	EVENING	BREAKFAST	MID MORN	LUNCH	AFTERNOON	DINNER	EVENING	BEDTIME
MONDAY											
TUESDAY											
WEDNESDAY											
THURSDAY											
FRIDAY											
SATURDAY											
SUNDAY											

NOTES

(Reasons for your blood glucose being high/low. Lack of exercise, sweets, carbs, alcohol etc.)

MONDAY:

TUESDAY:

WEDNESDAY:

THURSDAY:

FRIDAY:

SATURDAY:

SUNDAY:

DATE:	INSULIN UNITS				BLOOD GLUCOSE READING						
	BREAKFAST	LUNCH	DINNER	EVENING	BREAKFAST	MID MORN	LUNCH	AFTERNOON	DINNER	EVENING	BEDTIME
MONDAY											
TUESDAY											
WEDNESDAY											
THURSDAY											
FRIDAY											
SATURDAY											
SUNDAY											

NOTES

(Reasons for your blood glucose being high/low. Lack of exercise, sweets, carbs, alcohol etc.)

MONDAY:

TUESDAY:

WEDNESDAY:

THURSDAY:

FRIDAY:

SATURDAY:

SUNDAY:

DATE:	INSULIN UNITS				BLOOD GLUCOSE READING						
	BREAKFAST	LUNCH	DINNER	EVENING	BREAKFAST	MID MORN	LUNCH	AFTERNOON	DINNER	EVENING	BEDTIME
MONDAY											
TUESDAY											
WEDNESDAY											
THURSDAY											
FRIDAY											
SATURDAY											
SUNDAY											

NOTES

(Reasons for your blood glucose being high/low. Lack of exercise, sweets, carbs, alcohol etc.)

MONDAY:

TUESDAY:

WEDNESDAY:

THURSDAY:

FRIDAY:

SATURDAY:

SUNDAY:

DATE:	INSULIN UNITS				BLOOD GLUCOSE READING							
	BREAKFAST	LUNCH	DINNER	EVENING	BREAKFAST	MID MORN	LUNCH	AFTERNOON	DINNER	EVENING	BEDTIME
MONDAY											
TUESDAY											
WEDNESDAY											
THURSDAY											
FRIDAY											
SATURDAY											
SUNDAY											

NOTES
(Reasons for your blood glucose being high/low. Lack of exercise, sweets, carbs, alcohol etc.)

MONDAY:

TUESDAY:

WEDNESDAY:

THURSDAY:

FRIDAY:

SATURDAY:

SUNDAY:

DATE:	INSULIN UNITS				BLOOD GLUCOSE READING						
	BREAKFAST	LUNCH	DINNER	EVENING	BREAKFAST	MID MORN	LUNCH	AFTERNOON	DINNER	EVENING	BEDTIME
MONDAY											
TUESDAY											
WEDNESDAY											
THURSDAY											
FRIDAY											
SATURDAY											
SUNDAY											

NOTES

(Reasons for your blood glucose being high/low. Lack of exercise, sweets, carbs, alcohol etc.)

MONDAY:

TUESDAY:

WEDNESDAY:

THURSDAY:

FRIDAY:

SATURDAY:

SUNDAY:

DATE:		INSULIN UNITS				BLOOD GLUCOSE READING						
		BREAKFAST	LUNCH	DINNER	EVENING	BREAKFAST	MID MORN	LUNCH	AFTERNOON	DINNER	EVENING	BEDTIME
MONDAY												
TUESDAY												
WEDNESDAY												
THURSDAY												
FRIDAY												
SATURDAY												
SUNDAY												

NOTES
(Reasons for your blood glucose being high/low. Lack of exercise, sweets, carbs, alcohol etc.)

MONDAY:

TUESDAY:

WEDNESDAY:

THURSDAY:

FRIDAY:

SATURDAY:

SUNDAY:

DATE:	INSULIN UNITS				BLOOD GLUCOSE READING						
	BREAKFAST	LUNCH	DINNER	EVENING	BREAKFAST	MID MORN	LUNCH	AFTERNOON	DINNER	EVENING	BEDTIME
MONDAY											
TUESDAY											
WEDNESDAY											
THURSDAY											
FRIDAY											
SATURDAY											
SUNDAY											

NOTES

(Reasons for your blood glucose being high/low. Lack of exercise, sweets, carbs, alcohol etc.)

MONDAY:

TUESDAY:

WEDNESDAY:

THURSDAY:

FRIDAY:

SATURDAY:

SUNDAY:

DATE:	INSULIN UNITS				BLOOD GLUCOSE READING						
	BREAKFAST	LUNCH	DINNER	EVENING	BREAKFAST	MID MORN	LUNCH	AFTERNOON	DINNER	EVENING	BEDTIME
MONDAY											
TUESDAY											
WEDNESDAY											
THURSDAY											
FRIDAY											
SATURDAY											
SUNDAY											

NOTES

(Reasons for your blood glucose being high/low. Lack of exercise, sweets, carbs, alcohol etc.)

MONDAY:

TUESDAY:

WEDNESDAY:

THURSDAY:

FRIDAY:

SATURDAY:

SUNDAY:

DATE:	INSULIN UNITS				BLOOD GLUCOSE READING						
	BREAKFAST	LUNCH	DINNER	EVENING	BREAKFAST	MID MORN	LUNCH	AFTERNOON	DINNER	EVENING	BEDTIME
MONDAY											
TUESDAY											
WEDNESDAY											
THURSDAY											
FRIDAY											
SATURDAY											
SUNDAY											

NOTES
(Reasons for your blood glucose being high/low. Lack of exercise, sweets, carbs, alcohol etc.)

MONDAY:

TUESDAY:

WEDNESDAY:

THURSDAY:

FRIDAY:

SATURDAY:

SUNDAY:

DATE:	INSULIN UNITS				BLOOD GLUCOSE READING						
	BREAKFAST	LUNCH	DINNER	EVENING	BREAKFAST	MID MORN	LUNCH	AFTERNOON	DINNER	EVENING	BEDTIME
MONDAY											
TUESDAY											
WEDNESDAY											
THURSDAY											
FRIDAY											
SATURDAY											
SUNDAY											

NOTES

(Reasons for your blood glucose being high/low. Lack of exercise, sweets, carbs, alcohol etc.)

MONDAY:

TUESDAY:

WEDNESDAY:

THURSDAY:

FRIDAY:

SATURDAY:

SUNDAY:

DATE:	INSULIN UNITS				BLOOD GLUCOSE READING						
	B R E A K F A S T	L U N C H	D I N N E R	E V E N I N G	B R E A K F A S T	M I D M O R N	L U N C H	A F T E R N O O N	D I N N E R	E V E N I N G	B E D T I M E
MONDAY											
TUESDAY											
WEDNESDAY											
THURSDAY											
FRIDAY											
SATURDAY											
SUNDAY											

NOTES
(Reasons for your blood glucose being high/low. Lack of exercise, sweets, carbs, alcohol etc.)

MONDAY:

TUESDAY:

WEDNESDAY:

THURSDAY:

FRIDAY:

SATURDAY:

SUNDAY:

DATE:	INSULIN UNITS				BLOOD GLUCOSE READING						
	BREAKFAST	LUNCH	DINNER	EVENING	BREAKFAST	MID MORN	LUNCH	AFTERNOON	DINNER	EVENING	BEDTIME
MONDAY											
TUESDAY											
WEDNESDAY											
THURSDAY											
FRIDAY											
SATURDAY											
SUNDAY											

NOTES

(Reasons for your blood glucose being high/low. Lack of exercise, sweets, carbs, alcohol etc.)

MONDAY:

TUESDAY:

WEDNESDAY:

THURSDAY:

FRIDAY:

SATURDAY:

SUNDAY:

DATE:	INSULIN UNITS				BLOOD GLUCOSE READING						
	BREAKFAST	LUNCH	DINNER	EVENING	BREAKFAST	MID MORN	LUNCH	AFTERNOON	DINNER	EVENING	BEDTIME
MONDAY											
TUESDAY											
WEDNESDAY											
THURSDAY											
FRIDAY											
SATURDAY											
SUNDAY											

NOTES

(Reasons for your blood glucose being high/low. Lack of exercise, sweets, carbs, alcohol etc.)

MONDAY:

TUESDAY:

WEDNESDAY:

THURSDAY:

FRIDAY:

SATURDAY:

SUNDAY:

DATE:	INSULIN UNITS				BLOOD GLUCOSE READING						
	BREAKFAST	LUNCH	DINNER	EVENING	BREAKFAST	MID MORN	LUNCH	AFTERNOON	DINNER	EVENING	BEDTIME
MONDAY											
TUESDAY											
WEDNESDAY											
THURSDAY											
FRIDAY											
SATURDAY											
SUNDAY											

NOTES
(Reasons for your blood glucose being high/low. Lack of exercise, sweets, carbs, alcohol etc.)

MONDAY:

TUESDAY:

WEDNESDAY:

THURSDAY:

FRIDAY:

SATURDAY:

SUNDAY:

DATE:	INSULIN UNITS				BLOOD GLUCOSE READING						
	BREAKFAST	LUNCH	DINNER	EVENING	BREAKFAST	MID MORN	LUNCH	AFTERNOON	DINNER	EVENING	BEDTIME
MONDAY											
TUESDAY											
WEDNESDAY											
THURSDAY											
FRIDAY											
SATURDAY											
SUNDAY											

NOTES
(Reasons for your blood glucose being high/low. Lack of exercise, sweets, carbs, alcohol etc.)

MONDAY:

TUESDAY:

WEDNESDAY:

THURSDAY:

FRIDAY:

SATURDAY:

SUNDAY:

DATE:	INSULIN UNITS				BLOOD GLUCOSE READING							
	BREAKFAST	LUNCH	DINNER	EVENING	BREAKFAST	MID MORN	LUNCH	AFTERNOON	DINNER	EVENING	BEDTIME	
MONDAY												
TUESDAY												
WEDNESDAY												
THURSDAY												
FRIDAY												
SATURDAY												
SUNDAY												

NOTES
(Reasons for your blood glucose being high/low. Lack of exercise, sweets, carbs, alcohol etc.)

MONDAY:

TUESDAY:

WEDNESDAY:

THURSDAY:

FRIDAY:

SATURDAY:

SUNDAY:

DATE:	INSULIN UNITS				BLOOD GLUCOSE READING						
	BREAKFAST	LUNCH	DINNER	EVENING	BREAKFAST	MID MORN	LUNCH	AFTERNOON	DINNER	EVENING	BEDTIME
MONDAY											
TUESDAY											
WEDNESDAY											
THURSDAY											
FRIDAY											
SATURDAY											
SUNDAY											

NOTES

(Reasons for your blood glucose being high/low. Lack of exercise, sweets, carbs, alcohol etc.)

MONDAY:

TUESDAY:

WEDNESDAY:

THURSDAY:

FRIDAY:

SATURDAY:

SUNDAY:

DATE:	INSULIN UNITS				BLOOD GLUCOSE READING						
(clock image)	BREAKFAST	LUNCH	DINNER	EVENING	BREAKFAST	MID MORN	LUNCH	AFTERNOON	DINNER	EVENING	BEDTIME
MONDAY											
TUESDAY											
WEDNESDAY											
THURSDAY											
FRIDAY											
SATURDAY											
SUNDAY											

NOTES

(Reasons for your blood glucose being high/low. Lack of exercise, sweets, carbs, alcohol etc.)

MONDAY:

TUESDAY:

WEDNESDAY:

THURSDAY:

FRIDAY:

SATURDAY:

SUNDAY:

DATE:	INSULIN UNITS				BLOOD GLUCOSE READING							
	B R E A K F A S T	L U N C H	D I N N E R	E V E N I N G	B R E A K F A S T	M I D M O R N	L U N C H	A F T E R N O O N	D I N N E R	E V E N I N G	B E D T I M E
MONDAY											
TUESDAY											
WEDNESDAY											
THURSDAY											
FRIDAY											
SATURDAY											
SUNDAY											

NOTES

(Reasons for your blood glucose being high/low. Lack of exercise, sweets, carbs, alcohol etc.)

MONDAY:

TUESDAY:

WEDNESDAY:

THURSDAY:

FRIDAY:

SATURDAY:

SUNDAY:

DATE:	INSULIN UNITS				BLOOD GLUCOSE READING						
	BREAKFAST	LUNCH	DINNER	EVENING	BREAKFAST	MID MORN	LUNCH	AFTERNOON	DINNER	EVENING	BEDTIME
MONDAY											
TUESDAY											
WEDNESDAY											
THURSDAY											
FRIDAY											
SATURDAY											
SUNDAY											

NOTES

(Reasons for your blood glucose being high/low. Lack of exercise, sweets, carbs, alcohol etc.)

MONDAY:

TUESDAY:

WEDNESDAY:

THURSDAY:

FRIDAY:

SATURDAY:

SUNDAY:

DATE:	INSULIN UNITS				BLOOD GLUCOSE READING						
	BREAKFAST	LUNCH	DINNER	EVENING	BREAKFAST	MID MORN	LUNCH	AFTERNOON	DINNER	EVENING	BEDTIME
MONDAY											
TUESDAY											
WEDNESDAY											
THURSDAY											
FRIDAY											
SATURDAY											
SUNDAY											

<u>NOTES</u>

(Reasons for your blood glucose being high/low. Lack of exercise, sweets, carbs, alcohol etc.)

MONDAY:

TUESDAY:

WEDNESDAY:

THURSDAY:

FRIDAY:

SATURDAY:

SUNDAY:

DATE:	INSULIN UNITS				BLOOD GLUCOSE READING						
	BREAKFAST	LUNCH	DINNER	EVENING	BREAKFAST	MID MORN	LUNCH	AFTERNOON	DINNER	EVENING	BEDTIME
MONDAY											
TUESDAY											
WEDNESDAY											
THURSDAY											
FRIDAY											
SATURDAY											
SUNDAY											

NOTES
(Reasons for your blood glucose being high/low. Lack of exercise, sweets, carbs, alcohol etc.)

MONDAY:

TUESDAY:

WEDNESDAY:

THURSDAY:

FRIDAY:

SATURDAY:

SUNDAY:

DATE:	INSULIN UNITS				BLOOD GLUCOSE READING						
	BREAKFAST	LUNCH	DINNER	EVENING	BREAKFAST	MID MORN	LUNCH	AFTERNOON	DINNER	EVENING	BEDTIME
MONDAY											
TUESDAY											
WEDNESDAY											
THURSDAY											
FRIDAY											
SATURDAY											
SUNDAY											

NOTES

(Reasons for your blood glucose being high/low. Lack of exercise, sweets, carbs, alcohol etc.)

MONDAY:

TUESDAY:

WEDNESDAY:

THURSDAY:

FRIDAY:

SATURDAY:

SUNDAY:

DATE:	INSULIN UNITS				BLOOD GLUCOSE READING						
	BREAKFAST	LUNCH	DINNER	EVENING	BREAKFAST	MID MORN	LUNCH	AFTERNOON	DINNER	EVENING	BEDTIME
MONDAY											
TUESDAY											
WEDNESDAY											
THURSDAY											
FRIDAY											
SATURDAY											
SUNDAY											

NOTES

(Reasons for your blood glucose being high/low. Lack of exercise, sweets, carbs, alcohol etc.)

MONDAY:

TUESDAY:

WEDNESDAY:

THURSDAY:

FRIDAY:

SATURDAY:

SUNDAY:

DATE:	INSULIN UNITS				BLOOD GLUCOSE READING							
	BREAKFAST	LUNCH	DINNER	EVENING	BREAKFAST	MID MORN	LUNCH	AFTERNOON	DINNER	EVENING	BEDTIME
MONDAY											
TUESDAY											
WEDNESDAY											
THURSDAY											
FRIDAY											
SATURDAY											
SUNDAY											

NOTES

(Reasons for your blood glucose being high/low. Lack of exercise, sweets, carbs, alcohol etc.)

MONDAY:

TUESDAY:

WEDNESDAY:

THURSDAY:

FRIDAY:

SATURDAY:

SUNDAY:

DATE:	INSULIN UNITS				BLOOD GLUCOSE READING						
	BREAKFAST	LUNCH	DINNER	EVENING	BREAKFAST	MID MORN	LUNCH	AFTERNOON	DINNER	EVENING	BEDTIME
MONDAY											
TUESDAY											
WEDNESDAY											
THURSDAY											
FRIDAY											
SATURDAY											
SUNDAY											

NOTES
(Reasons for your blood glucose being high/low. Lack of exercise, sweets, carbs, alcohol etc.)

MONDAY:

TUESDAY:

WEDNESDAY:

THURSDAY:

FRIDAY:

SATURDAY:

SUNDAY:

DATE:	INSULIN UNITS				BLOOD GLUCOSE READING						
	BREAKFAST	LUNCH	DINNER	EVENING	BREAKFAST	MID MORN	LUNCH	AFTERNOON	DINNER	EVENING	BEDTIME
MONDAY											
TUESDAY											
WEDNESDAY											
THURSDAY											
FRIDAY											
SATURDAY											
SUNDAY											

NOTES
(Reasons for your blood glucose being high/low. Lack of exercise, sweets, carbs, alcohol etc.)

MONDAY:

TUESDAY:

WEDNESDAY:

THURSDAY:

FRIDAY:

SATURDAY:

SUNDAY:

DATE:	INSULIN UNITS				BLOOD GLUCOSE READING						
	BREAKFAST	LUNCH	DINNER	EVENING	BREAKFAST	MID MORN	LUNCH	AFTERNOON	DINNER	EVENING	BEDTIME
MONDAY											
TUESDAY											
WEDNESDAY											
THURSDAY											
FRIDAY											
SATURDAY											
SUNDAY											

NOTES

(Reasons for your blood glucose being high/low. Lack of exercise, sweets, carbs, alcohol etc.)

MONDAY:

TUESDAY:

WEDNESDAY:

THURSDAY:

FRIDAY:

SATURDAY:

SUNDAY:

DATE:	INSULIN UNITS				BLOOD GLUCOSE READING						
(clock)	BREAKFAST	LUNCH	DINNER	EVENING	BREAKFAST	MID MORN	LUNCH	AFTERNOON	DINNER	EVENING	BEDTIME
MONDAY											
TUESDAY											
WEDNESDAY											
THURSDAY											
FRIDAY											
SATURDAY											
SUNDAY											

NOTES

(Reasons for your blood glucose being high/low. Lack of exercise, sweets, carbs, alcohol etc.)

MONDAY:

TUESDAY:

WEDNESDAY:

THURSDAY:

FRIDAY:

SATURDAY:

SUNDAY:

DATE:	INSULIN UNITS				BLOOD GLUCOSE READING						
⏰	BREAKFAST	LUNCH	DINNER	EVENING	BREAKFAST	MID MORN	LUNCH	AFTERNOON	DINNER	EVENING	BEDTIME
MONDAY											
TUESDAY											
WEDNESDAY											
THURSDAY											
FRIDAY											
SATURDAY											
SUNDAY											

NOTES

(Reasons for your blood glucose being high/low. Lack of exercise, sweets, carbs, alcohol etc.)

MONDAY:

TUESDAY:

WEDNESDAY:

THURSDAY:

FRIDAY:

SATURDAY:

SUNDAY:

DATE:	INSULIN UNITS				BLOOD GLUCOSE READING						
	BREAKFAST	LUNCH	DINNER	EVENING	BREAKFAST	MID MORN	LUNCH	AFTERNOON	DINNER	EVENING	BEDTIME
MONDAY											
TUESDAY											
WEDNESDAY											
THURSDAY											
FRIDAY											
SATURDAY											
SUNDAY											

NOTES
(Reasons for your blood glucose being high/low. Lack of exercise, sweets, carbs, alcohol etc.)

MONDAY:

TUESDAY:

WEDNESDAY:

THURSDAY:

FRIDAY:

SATURDAY:

SUNDAY:

DATE:	INSULIN UNITS				BLOOD GLUCOSE READING							
	BREAKFAST	LUNCH	DINNER	EVENING	BREAKFAST	MID MORN	LUNCH	AFTERNOON	DINNER	EVENING	BEDTIME
MONDAY											
TUESDAY											
WEDNESDAY											
THURSDAY											
FRIDAY											
SATURDAY											
SUNDAY											

NOTES

(Reasons for your blood glucose being high/low. Lack of exercise, sweets, carbs, alcohol etc.)

MONDAY:

TUESDAY:

WEDNESDAY:

THURSDAY:

FRIDAY:

SATURDAY:

SUNDAY:

DATE:	INSULIN UNITS				BLOOD GLUCOSE READING						
	BREAKFAST	LUNCH	DINNER	EVENING	BREAKFAST	MID MORN	LUNCH	AFTERNOON	DINNER	EVENING	BEDTIME
MONDAY											
TUESDAY											
WEDNESDAY											
THURSDAY											
FRIDAY											
SATURDAY											
SUNDAY											

NOTES
(Reasons for your blood glucose being high/low. Lack of exercise, sweets, carbs, alcohol etc.)

MONDAY:

TUESDAY:

WEDNESDAY:

THURSDAY:

FRIDAY:

SATURDAY:

SUNDAY:

DATE:	INSULIN UNITS				BLOOD GLUCOSE READING						
	BREAKFAST	LUNCH	DINNER	EVENING	BREAKFAST	MID MORN	LUNCH	AFTERNOON	DINNER	EVENING	BEDTIME
MONDAY											
TUESDAY											
WEDNESDAY											
THURSDAY											
FRIDAY											
SATURDAY											
SUNDAY											

NOTES
(Reasons for your blood glucose being high/low. Lack of exercise, sweets, carbs, alcohol etc.)

MONDAY:

TUESDAY:

WEDNESDAY:

THURSDAY:

FRIDAY:

SATURDAY:

SUNDAY:

DATE:	INSULIN UNITS				BLOOD GLUCOSE READING						
	BREAKFAST	LUNCH	DINNER	EVENING	BREAKFAST	MID MORN	LUNCH	AFTERNOON	DINNER	EVENING	BEDTIME
MONDAY											
TUESDAY											
WEDNESDAY											
THURSDAY											
FRIDAY											
SATURDAY											
SUNDAY											

NOTES

(Reasons for your blood glucose being high/low. Lack of exercise, sweets, carbs, alcohol etc.)

MONDAY:

TUESDAY:

WEDNESDAY:

THURSDAY:

FRIDAY:

SATURDAY:

SUNDAY:

DATE:	INSULIN UNITS				BLOOD GLUCOSE READING						
	BREAKFAST	LUNCH	DINNER	EVENING	BREAKFAST	MID MORN	LUNCH	AFTERNOON	DINNER	EVENING	BEDTIME
MONDAY											
TUESDAY											
WEDNESDAY											
THURSDAY											
FRIDAY											
SATURDAY											
SUNDAY											

NOTES
(Reasons for your blood glucose being high/low. Lack of exercise, sweets, carbs, alcohol etc.)

MONDAY:

TUESDAY:

WEDNESDAY:

THURSDAY:

FRIDAY:

SATURDAY:

SUNDAY: